LUPUS UNCOVERED

Essential Insights and Practical Guidance for Patients

Pete Gregory, MD

TABLE OF CONTENTS

Contents

TABLE OF CONTENTS 1
CHAPTER 1: UNDERSTANDING LUPUS 2
    Overview of Lupus 3
    Types of Lupus and Their Differences 4
    The Autoimmune Nature of Lupus 7
CHAPTER 2: RECOGNIZING THE SYMPTOMS OF LUPUS 10
    Common Signs and Symptoms 11
    How Lupus Affects Different Organs 15
    When to Seek Medical Help 17
CHAPTER 3: DIAGNOSING LUPUS 21
    How Lupus is Diagnosed 22
    Blood Tests and Other Diagnostic Tools 23
    The Importance of Early Detection 27
CHAPTER 4: MANAGING LUPUS FLARE-UPS 31
    What Causes Flare-Ups? 32
    How to Spot a Flare-Up 34
    Coping Strategies During a Flare-Up 36
CHAPTER 5: TREATMENT OPTIONS FOR LUPUS 40
    Medications Used in Lupus Treatment 41

Understanding Steroids, Immunosuppressants, and Biologics ... 44

Alternative and Complementary Therapies ... 46

CHAPTER 6: LIVING WITH LUPUS ... 50

Managing Fatigue and Pain ... 51

Adapting Your Routine for Better Health ... 53

Protecting Your Skin and Sun Safety ... 56

CHAPTER 7: NUTRITION AND LUPUS ... 59

The Role of Diet in Lupus Management ... 60

Foods to Include and Avoid ... 62

Supplements and Nutritional Support ... 67

CHAPTER 8: EXERCISE AND PHYSICAL ACTIVITY WITH LUPUS ... 71

Benefits of Staying Active ... 72

Choosing the Right Exercise Routine ... 74

How to Exercise Safely During a Flare-Up ... 77

CHAPTER 9: EMOTIONAL HEALTH AND COPING WITH LUPUS ... 82

The Mental and Emotional Impact of Lupus ... 83

Coping with Anxiety and Depression ... 85

Building a Support System ... 88

CHAPTER 10: THE ROLE OF YOUR HEALTHCARE TEAM ... 92

Why Working with Your Doctors is Important ... 93

How to Build a Good Care Plan ... 96

When to Get a Second Opinion ... 99

CHAPTER 11: PREGNANCY AND LUPUS ... 103

Managing Lupus During Pregnancy ... 104

Risks and Precautions for Expecting Mothers ... 106

Postpartum Considerations for Lupus Patients ... 109

CHAPTER 12: LUPUS AND WORK ... 113

Navigating Work with Lupus ... 114

Communicating with Your Employer ... 117

Legal Rights and Protections for Lupus Patients ... 120

CHAPTER 13: LOOKING AHEAD ... 123

Setting Goals for Your Health Journey ... 123

Preventing Complications and Managing Risks ... 126

Embracing a Positive Outlook and Living Your Best Life ... 129

Thank You! ... 133

A Personal Note ... 134

The Power of Knowledge ... 135

Acknowledging the Challenges ... 137

The Importance of Community and Support ... 139

Looking Forward ... 140

CHAPTER 1: UNDERSTANDING LUPUS

Lupus is a disease where the body's immune system, which usually protects us from infections, starts attacking the body's healthy tissues by mistake. This can cause pain and swelling in different parts of the body like the skin, joints, kidneys, heart, and lungs. While doctors don't know exactly what causes lupus, they believe a mix of genes (the things that make us who we are) and things from the environment, like sunlight or infections, might trigger it. Learning about lupus can help people with the disease manage it better and live a healthier life.

Overview of Lupus

Lupus is an autoimmune disease. This means the immune system, instead of helping protect the body, attacks it by mistake. This causes inflammation and pain in different parts of the body. Sometimes lupus can affect just one area, but other times it can hurt many parts of the body at once. Symptoms of lupus are not the same for everyone. Some people have mild symptoms, like joint pain or a rash, while others might experience more serious issues, like kidney problems. These symptoms can come and go, with some people having flare-ups where symptoms get worse, and others feeling better for a while.

There are also things that can cause lupus to flare up, like stress, infections, certain medicines, or too much sun. But doctors don't fully understand why lupus happens, so they're still researching it to find better treatments and maybe even a cure someday.

Types of Lupus and Their Differences

While lupus usually refers to a type called systemic lupus erythematosus (SLE), which is the most common and serious form, there are other types of lupus that affect the body in different ways:

1. Systemic Lupus Erythematosus (SLE) SLE is the most common type and can affect many parts of the body, including the skin, kidneys, joints, and heart. Some people might only have mild symptoms, like a butterfly-shaped rash across their face or joint pain, while others might have more serious problems.

2. Discoid Lupus Erythematosus (DLE) DLE mostly affects the skin, causing red, scaly patches that can lead to scarring or hair loss. It doesn't affect internal organs like SLE, and it may come and go in flare-ups.

3. Drug-Induced Lupus Some medicines can cause symptoms that

look like lupus. This is called drug-induced lupus, and it usually goes away once the medicine is stopped. It tends to be milder than SLE and doesn't cause as much damage to organs.

4. Neonatal Lupus Neonatal lupus is a rare type that affects newborn babies. It happens when certain antibodies from the mother pass through to the baby during pregnancy. The baby may have a rash or heart problems, but these symptoms usually go away after a few months.

5. Subacute Cutaneous Lupus Erythematosus (SCLE) SCLE mainly affects the skin and causes rashes, especially after sun exposure. It can

also sometimes affect internal organs, though not as much as SLE. People with SCLE may also develop SLE over time.

The Autoimmune Nature of Lupus

Lupus is an autoimmune disease, which means the body's immune system starts attacking its own healthy tissues. Normally, the immune system fights infections, but in lupus, it mistakenly targets the body's own cells. This causes inflammation, pain, and damage to different parts of the body. No one really knows why the immune system makes this mistake, but both genetics (what you inherit from your parents) and things in the environment, like infections or stress, may trigger lupus. Lupus is more common in women, especially those in their childbearing years, which suggests that hormones might play a role too.

Doctors treat lupus by trying to control the immune system, so it doesn't attack the body. This is usually done with medications that reduce the inflammation and calm the immune system, like steroids and other immune-suppressing drugs.

Conclusion

Lupus is a disease that can affect many parts of the body, but it's different for everyone. While there is no cure yet, there are treatments that help people manage their symptoms and live better lives. By understanding the different types of lupus, how the immune system causes it, and the things that can trigger it, people with lupus can work with their doctors to make a plan for managing it. Learning about lupus can help people take charge of their health and live full lives, even with the disease.

CHAPTER 2: RECOGNIZING THE SYMPTOMS OF LUPUS

Lupus is a tricky disease that can affect many parts of your body, and its symptoms can be different for each person. It can be hard to recognize because the signs may look like other illnesses. But catching it early can help you manage it better and live a healthier life. This chapter explains the common symptoms of lupus, how it affects different organs in your body, and when you should see a doctor.

Common Signs and Symptoms

The symptoms of lupus can start out mild but may get worse over time. It happens when the body's immune system attacks its own tissues, causing inflammation. Some of the most common signs of lupus include:

1. Fatigue (Tiredness): One of the most common symptoms of lupus is feeling very tired all the time, even after a full night of sleep. You may feel worn out for no reason, and this tiredness can make it hard to do normal activities.

2. Joint Pain and Swelling: Many people with lupus feel pain, swelling,

and stiffness in their joints, especially in the hands, wrists, and knees. This can make it difficult to move, and it can feel a lot like arthritis, but not as severe.

3. Butterfly Rash: A common sign of lupus is a rash shaped like a butterfly that appears on the cheeks and nose. It can look red or purple and often gets worse when you are out in the sun.

4. Sensitivity to Sunlight (Photosensitivity): People with lupus often get a rash or flare-ups if they spend time in the sun. Sunlight can make their symptoms worse, so it's important to protect the skin.

5. Hair Loss: Lupus can cause your hair to thin or fall out, especially during flare-ups. Your hair may grow back when the disease is under control.

6. Mouth and Nose Sores: People with lupus often get sores inside their mouth or nose. These sores don't usually hurt but can be annoying, especially when eating or talking.

7. Chest Pain and Shortness of Breath: If lupus affects your heart or lungs, it can cause chest pain or make it hard to breathe. This happens when the inflammation affects the heart lining (pericarditis) or the lungs (pleuritis).

8. Raynaud's Phenomenon: This condition causes fingers and toes to turn white or blue when it's cold or stressful. It happens because the small blood vessels in your hands and feet tighten and stop the blood from flowing properly.

9. Fever: Sometimes people with lupus get a low fever, even when there's no infection. This usually happens during flare-ups when the immune system is more active.

How Lupus Affects Different Organs

Lupus is called a "systemic" disease because it can affect many parts of the body at once. Here's how lupus can impact different organs:

1. Skin: Lupus can cause rashes, sores, and skin problems, especially on the face, neck, and arms. People with lupus are also more sensitive to the sun, which can make the skin problems worse.

2. Joints: Lupus can cause joint pain, swelling, and stiffness. This can make it hard to move, and over time, if not treated, it can lead to joint problems.

3. Kidneys: Sometimes lupus affects the kidneys, which can cause swelling in the legs, ankles, or feet, and make you have to pee more or less than usual. If not treated, lupus can lead to kidney failure.

4. Heart: Lupus can cause inflammation in the heart or its lining, leading to chest pain, difficulty breathing, and an increased risk of heart problems.

5. Lungs: Lupus can cause inflammation in the lungs, making it hard to breathe and causing chest pain or coughing. In severe cases, it can cause scarring in the lungs.

6. Brain and Nervous System: Lupus can also affect the brain, causing headaches, memory problems, mood changes, or even seizures.

When to Seek Medical Help

Lupus can be hard to diagnose because its symptoms are similar to those of other diseases. If you notice any of the common symptoms of lupus, you should see a doctor. Early treatment can prevent long-term damage and help you feel better.

You should see a doctor if you have:

A rash, especially a butterfly-shaped rash on your face

Pain, swelling, or stiffness in your joints

A fever that lasts for a few days

Feeling very tired, even after rest

Trouble breathing, chest pain, or shortness of breath

Severe headaches, memory loss, or mood changes

Swelling in your legs, feet, or ankles, or changes in how often you pee

Sensitivity to the sun that makes your symptoms worse

If you already know you have lupus and any of these symptoms happen, it's important to contact your doctor right away. A lupus flare-up can cause serious problems, and catching it early can help prevent further damage.

Conclusion

Lupus affects different parts of your body and can cause many symptoms. Recognizing the signs of lupus early can help you get treatment and prevent serious health problems. If you notice any of the symptoms we talked about, or if your symptoms get worse, don't hesitate to see a doctor. Working with your healthcare team to manage your symptoms can help you live a happy, healthy life despite lupus. By understanding the signs of lupus, you can take control of your health and feel more confident managing the disease.

CHAPTER 3: DIAGNOSING LUPUS

Lupus is a tricky disease that is hard to diagnose. Its symptoms can be similar to other illnesses, making it difficult for doctors to figure out right away. But if you understand how lupus is diagnosed, the tests used to find it, and why it's important to catch it early, it can help you get the right diagnosis and treatment. This chapter will explain how doctors figure out if you have lupus, the tests they use, and why it's important to find it early.

How Lupus is Diagnosed

Diagnosing lupus isn't simple. There isn't one test or symptom that can tell for sure if you have lupus, and many of its signs are similar to other diseases. That's why doctors look at many different things to make a diagnosis, including your medical history, symptoms, physical exam, and tests.

When you first go to the doctor, they will ask about your symptoms, like when they started and how they've changed. Since lupus can affect many parts of your body, they'll also ask about things like joint pain, tiredness, rashes, or chest pain. During your exam, the doctor will look for signs of lupus, like the butterfly-shaped rash that appears on the face or swollen joints.

But because lupus can look like other diseases, doctors need more information to be sure. That's where tests and scans come in. There isn't one test that can tell for sure if you have lupus, but there are many tests that can help doctors figure it out. The results of these tests, along with your symptoms and exam, will help the doctor decide if you have lupus.

Blood Tests and Other Diagnostic Tools

Blood tests are very important for diagnosing lupus. One common test is the antinuclear antibody (ANA) test, which checks if your body is making antibodies that attack your own cells. If your ANA test is positive, it might suggest lupus, but it's not certain because some healthy people can also have a positive ANA test. The ANA test is usually just the starting point, and your doctor will likely do other tests to get more information.

1. Anti-dsDNA and Anti-Sm Antibodies: These are more specific tests for lupus. If your blood has anti-dsDNA antibodies, it's a strong sign that you may have lupus, especially a type called systemic lupus erythematosus (SLE). Another test for anti-Sm antibodies also helps confirm lupus.

2. Complete Blood Count (CBC): This test looks at the number of red blood cells, white blood cells, and platelets in your blood. Lupus can cause low red blood cells (anemia), white blood cells, or platelets, which can be a sign of the disease.

3. Urine Tests: Urine tests check if your kidneys are being affected by lupus. If your urine has protein or blood in it, this can mean lupus is harming your kidneys.

4. Complement Levels: These are proteins that help your body fight infections. In lupus, these levels can be lower, especially when the disease is more active.

5. ESR and CRP: These tests check for signs of inflammation in your body. When lupus is active, your inflammation levels might be high, even if you don't feel sick right away.

6. Imaging Studies: Tests like X-rays or ultrasounds can be used to see if lupus has caused damage to organs like your joints, heart, or lungs. These scans help doctors understand how lupus is affecting your body.

It's important to know that no single test can confirm lupus. Doctors use a combination of these tests and your symptoms to make a diagnosis. The tests help build a picture of whether you have lupus or not.

The Importance of Early Detection

Finding lupus early is really important for several reasons. First, when lupus is diagnosed early, it's easier to treat before it causes serious damage to organs like the kidneys, heart, or lungs. Lupus is a disease that can change quickly, with symptoms getting better or worse without warning. If it isn't treated, it can damage your organs over time.

When lupus is diagnosed early, treatment can start right away.

Treatment usually involves medicines that help calm the immune system and reduce swelling. Medications like corticosteroids, antimalarial drugs, and immunosuppressants help control symptoms and prevent long-term damage. The sooner you start treatment, the better your chances of feeling better and avoiding big problems later on.

Early detection also helps with managing the symptoms of lupus, like joint pain, skin rashes, and tiredness. While these symptoms aren't usually life-threatening, they can make daily life harder. If you catch lupus early, you can often reduce these symptoms and continue living an active life.

Plus, finding lupus early helps you keep track of your health. Regular checkups, blood tests, and scans can make sure that your lupus is under control and that any problems are caught early. Early detection also means you can learn more about lupus and take charge of your health by making better choices about treatment and self-care.

Conclusion

Diagnosing lupus isn't simple, but with the right tests and a careful look at your symptoms, doctors can figure out if you have it and start treatment. Blood tests, physical exams, and scans all help doctors make an accurate diagnosis. Catching lupus early is important because it helps you start treatment faster, manage symptoms better, and prevent serious damage to your organs. If you think you might have lupus or have symptoms that worry you, it's important to see a doctor as soon as possible. Knowing how lupus is diagnosed and why early detection matters can help you take the first step toward feeling better and managing your health.

CHAPTER 4: MANAGING LUPUS FLARE-UPS

Lupus is a disease that can cause sudden flare-ups, where your symptoms get worse all of a sudden. These flare-ups can be tough to handle, but by understanding what causes them, how to spot them early, and ways to manage them, you can take better control of your condition. This chapter will help you learn what triggers flare-ups, how to recognize when they're happening, and how to deal with them.

What Causes Flare-Ups?

Flare-ups happen when certain things trigger your lupus and make your symptoms worse. These triggers can be different for everyone, but some common ones include:

1. Sun Exposure: Being in the sun too long can cause your lupus symptoms to flare up. Sunlight can make your immune system overreact, causing skin problems or other issues in your body.

2. Stress: When you're stressed out, whether it's from school, friends, or home life, it can make your lupus worse. Stress can make your immune

system go into overdrive, which can lead to flare-ups.

3. Infections: If you get sick with something like a cold or an infection, your immune system gets activated, which can trigger a flare-up.

4. Medications: Some medicines can make lupus flare-ups worse, especially those that affect your immune system.

5. Hormonal Changes: Changes in hormones, like during puberty, menstruation, or pregnancy, can also cause flare-ups.

6. Environmental Factors: Things like extreme weather, pollution, or chemicals in the air can trigger flare-ups too. For example, cold weather can make your hands and feet feel numb.

How to Spot a Flare-Up

Knowing when a flare-up is starting can help you deal with it before it gets worse. Flare-ups can happen suddenly or build up over time, and some signs to look for include:

1. Feeling Extra Tired: If you suddenly feel more tired than usual, even though you haven't been doing anything extra, it could be a sign of a flare-up.

2. Joint Pain and Swelling: Your joints, like your hands and knees, might hurt or swell more than usual during a flare-up.

3. Skin Changes: A red rash that looks like a butterfly on your face is common in lupus. If your rash gets worse, or if you notice new rashes after being in the sun, it might be a flare.

4. Fever: If you feel hot or get a low fever (higher than 100°F), it could mean your lupus is flaring up.

5. Chest Pain or Trouble Breathing: If you feel pain in your chest or have trouble breathing, it could mean lupus

is affecting your heart or lungs, and you should get medical help right away.

6. Headaches and Trouble Focusing: During a flare, you might get headaches or have trouble thinking clearly. This is sometimes called "lupus fog."

Coping Strategies During a Flare-Up

When a flare-up happens, there are things you can do to make yourself feel better and manage the symptoms:

1. Stick to Your Treatment: Make sure you take your medicines as prescribed.

If you're not sure about something, ask your doctor. This helps to control your symptoms and prevent the flare from getting worse.

2. Rest and Save Your Energy: When you feel tired, rest! Don't push yourself too hard. Taking naps or lying down can help your body heal and keep your immune system from getting more stressed.

3. Reduce Stress: Since stress makes lupus worse, find ways to relax. Try deep breathing, listening to music, or talking to someone you trust. Taking time to do things you enjoy can also help.

4. Avoid the Sun: Since sunlight can make lupus flare-ups worse, stay in the shade or wear protective clothes, like a hat and sunscreen, if you have to go outside.

5. Track Your Symptoms: Keep track of how you're feeling. Write down any changes in your symptoms, the medicines you take, and what you think might be causing the flare-up. This can help you and your doctor figure out what works best for you.

6. Get Support: It can be hard to go through a flare-up on your own. Talk to family or friends who understand what you're going through. There are also

support groups online or in person where you can connect with others who have lupus.

Conclusion

Managing lupus flare-ups means knowing what causes them, recognizing the signs early, and using strategies to cope. By following your treatment plan, resting when you need to, and reducing stress, you can help prevent flare-ups from getting worse. Although flare-ups can be tough, they're a part of living with lupus, and with the right tools, you can manage them and continue with your life.

CHAPTER 5: TREATMENT OPTIONS FOR LUPUS

Lupus is a disease where the body's immune system attacks its own healthy tissues. There's no cure for lupus, but there are many ways to treat it and help manage the symptoms. The treatment plan depends on how severe the lupus is and which parts of the body it affects. In this chapter, we will look at the medicines used to treat lupus, the role of steroids, immune-suppressing drugs, and biologics, and also some alternative treatments that can help.

Medications Used in Lupus Treatment

Several types of medicines help control lupus symptoms. Some medicines reduce inflammation (swelling and redness), while others make the immune system weaker so it doesn't attack the body as much. A doctor will often use a combination of medicines to treat lupus.

1. NSAIDs (Nonsteroidal Anti-inflammatory Drugs): These medicines, like ibuprofen and naproxen, are used to reduce pain and swelling. They help with joint pain, muscle aches, and other mild symptoms of lupus. However, using them for a long time can cause problems with the kidneys or stomach.

2. Antimalarial Drugs: Hydroxychloroquine (Plaquenil) is a medicine originally used to treat malaria, but it is also very helpful for lupus. It helps with skin rashes, joint pain, and can reduce the chance of lupus flare-ups. It's one of the most common treatments for lupus.

3. Corticosteroids (Steroids): These are strong medicines used during a lupus flare-up to reduce swelling and pain. Prednisone is the most common steroid for lupus. It works quickly to control symptoms, but using steroids for a long time can cause problems like weight gain, weaker bones, high blood pressure, and more. Doctors try to use

the lowest dose possible to avoid these problems.

4. Immunosuppressive Drugs: These medicines make the immune system weaker so it doesn't attack the body. They are used for more serious cases of lupus when organs like the kidneys, heart, or lungs are affected. These drugs can be helpful but can also make it harder for the body to fight infections and may cause other side effects.

5. Biologic Therapies: These are newer treatments for lupus that target specific parts of the immune system. For example, belimumab (Benlysta) helps reduce lupus activity by stopping a protein that causes the immune system

to attack the body. Biologics are usually used when other treatments haven't worked well.

Understanding Steroids, Immunosuppressants, and Biologics

1. Steroids (Corticosteroids): Steroids are very effective at controlling symptoms of lupus, but doctors usually only give them for short periods because of the possible side effects. Long-term use can cause problems, so doctors try to lower the dose as soon as the flare-up is under control.

2. Immunosuppressants: These medicines stop the immune system from attacking healthy tissues. They are used for more severe lupus cases and can be helpful, but they also make the body more likely to get infections. Some immunosuppressive drugs can also cause liver problems or affect fertility.

3. Biologics: Biologics work by targeting specific parts of the immune system that cause lupus. These treatments are newer and help reduce flare-ups. They are used if other treatments haven't worked. Biologics are given through an injection or IV, but they also need careful monitoring because they can increase the risk of infections.

Alternative and Complementary Therapies

Besides regular medicines, some people with lupus try other treatments to help with symptoms. These treatments should not replace prescribed medicines, but they may help improve overall health and well-being. It's important to talk to a doctor before trying any new treatments.

1. Diet and Nutrition: Eating a healthy diet is very important for people with lupus. Some foods can make lupus symptoms worse, while others can help reduce inflammation. Eating fruits, vegetables, and foods with omega-3 fatty acids (like fish) can help lower inflammation. Avoiding too much

sugar, processed foods, and unhealthy fats is also a good idea.

2. Exercise: Regular exercise helps keep the body strong and healthy. Gentle activities like walking, swimming, or yoga can help with joint pain and improve flexibility. Exercise also helps with tiredness, a common symptom of lupus. However, it's important not to push yourself too hard during a flare-up.

3. Acupuncture: Some people find relief from pain and inflammation with acupuncture. This is a treatment where thin needles are inserted into certain points on the body. It can help manage pain, reduce stress, and improve

circulation, but more research is needed to prove how well it works for lupus.

4. Herbal Remedies: Some herbs, like turmeric, ginger, and fish oil, are thought to help reduce inflammation. However, it's important to talk to a doctor before using any herbal remedies because they can interact with medicines or cause side effects.

5. Mind-Body Practices: Stress can trigger lupus flare-ups, so learning to manage stress is important. Techniques like meditation, deep breathing, and relaxation exercises can help reduce stress and improve mental health.

Conclusion

While there is no cure for lupus, there are many ways to treat it and control symptoms. Medicines like steroids, immunosuppressants, and biologics are used to manage flare-ups, reduce inflammation, and prevent damage to organs. Additionally, alternative therapies like a healthy diet, exercise, acupuncture, and stress management can help improve quality of life. It's important to work with your doctor to create a treatment plan that's right for you. With the right care, people with lupus can live active and fulfilling lives.

CHAPTER 6: LIVING WITH LUPUS

Lupus is a long-term illness where the body's immune system attacks its own tissues. It can affect different parts of the body, making everyday activities harder. Although there is no cure for lupus, there are ways to manage the symptoms and live a good life. In this chapter, we'll talk about how to handle fatigue and pain, adjust your routine for better health, and keep your skin safe from the sun.

Managing Fatigue and Pain

Fatigue (feeling really tired) and pain are two of the most common and hardest symptoms of lupus. Many people with lupus feel tired all the time, even after sleeping a full night. Pain, especially in the joints and muscles, can also be a problem. These symptoms can make everyday activities feel harder and may cause stress. But with the right steps, it's possible to manage these problems and live well.

1. Get Enough Rest and Sleep: Fatigue is a common symptom of lupus, so getting enough sleep is very important. Try to get 7-9 hours of sleep each night. If you have trouble sleeping, try creating a bedtime routine to help you

relax, like avoiding caffeine or heavy meals before bed. Napping during the day can also help if you're feeling extra tired, especially during a lupus flare-up.

2. Don't Overdo It: It's important to take breaks and not do too much. Split up bigger tasks into smaller ones and take regular breaks. Listen to your body—if you feel tired, stop and rest. Do your hardest tasks when you have the most energy, and save easier tasks for later.

3. Pain Relief: Pain is another big part of lupus. Medicines like ibuprofen can help with joint and muscle pain. But be careful about using them too much, and talk to your doctor to find the right treatment for your pain. When pain gets worse, doctors might prescribe stronger

medicines. Physical therapy and gentle exercise can also help reduce pain by strengthening muscles and joints. Heat or cold packs, acupuncture, and massage therapy can sometimes offer extra help with pain.

Adapting Your Routine for Better Health

Changing your daily routine can help you feel better and avoid flare-ups. Small changes in your lifestyle can have a big impact on your health. Having a routine that includes taking care of your health, eating well, managing stress, and getting some exercise can help you feel better and keep lupus under control.

1. Stick to a Medication Schedule: Taking your prescribed medicines on time is really important for managing lupus. This could include steroids, medicines to suppress the immune system, or other drugs. Using a pill organizer or setting alarms on your phone can help you remember when to take your medicine. This helps prevent flare-ups and keeps lupus from getting worse.

2. Eat Healthy: What you eat matters when you have lupus. Eating fruits, vegetables, whole grains, and foods with omega-3 fats (like fish and nuts) can help reduce inflammation. Try to avoid processed foods, sugar, and too much salt, as these can trigger flare-ups. You might want to talk to a

nutritionist to make a meal plan that's best for you.

3. Exercise, but Don't Overdo It: Exercise is good for people with lupus, but it's important to avoid pushing yourself too hard. Low-impact exercises like walking, swimming, or yoga are great for helping your body stay strong without causing pain. Start with short exercise sessions and slowly increase the time you spend being active. Regular exercise can help with mood, energy, and reducing fatigue.

4. Manage Stress: Stress can make lupus worse, so it's important to find ways to relax. Try deep breathing exercises, meditation, or journaling to help reduce stress. Set aside some time each day to relax, even if it's just for a

few minutes. Having a strong support system, like friends, family, or support groups, can also help you feel better emotionally.

Protecting Your Skin and Sun Safety

Lupus can make your skin more sensitive to the sun, which can cause rashes or flare-ups. Protecting your skin from the sun is very important to prevent damage and keep your skin healthy.

1. Use Sunscreen Every Day: Sunscreen is essential for everyone with lupus. The sun's rays can make lupus worse and cause rashes. Use

sunscreen with an SPF of at least 30, and apply it to all exposed skin, even when it's cloudy. Reapply every two hours if you're outside or swimming. Look for sunscreens that are fragrance-free and made for sensitive skin.

2. Stay in the Shade and Avoid the Sun: Besides using sunscreen, it's important to stay out of direct sunlight. Try to stay in the shade, especially between 10 a.m. and 4 p.m., when the sun is strongest. Wearing hats, sunglasses, and long sleeves can help protect your skin from harmful UV rays.

3. Check Your Skin Regularly: People with lupus should keep an eye on their skin for any changes, like rashes or blisters. If you notice anything unusual,

talk to your doctor. Early treatment can prevent problems from getting worse.

Conclusion

Living with lupus can be tough, but with the right strategies, you can manage the symptoms and live a full life. Managing fatigue and pain, adjusting your daily routine, and protecting your skin are all important steps in living well with lupus. Take care of your body, stay on top of your medications, and make time for relaxation and support. By making small changes and staying proactive in your lupus care, you can improve your health and reduce how much lupus affects your daily life.

CHAPTER 7: NUTRITION AND LUPUS

When you have lupus, it's really important to eat the right foods to help manage your condition. Lupus is a disease where your immune system attacks your own body, causing inflammation and different health problems. While eating healthy won't cure lupus, the right diet can help reduce symptoms, prevent flare-ups, and keep you feeling better overall. This chapter will talk about how food affects lupus, what foods are good for you, and which ones to avoid.

The Role of Diet in Lupus Management

The food you eat can play a big part in how you feel when you have lupus. Eating the right foods helps keep your immune system in check, reduce inflammation, and give you the energy you need.

1. Reducing Inflammation: Lupus causes inflammation in the body, which can make you feel tired and in pain. Some foods make inflammation worse, while others can help reduce it. Foods like processed snacks and sugary treats can make inflammation worse, while

fruits, vegetables, and healthy fats can help calm it down.
*

2. Supporting the Immune System: Since lupus affects your immune system, eating foods with the right vitamins and minerals can help keep your immune system working properly, so it doesn't attack your healthy tissues.

3. Managing Other Health Problems: Lupus often comes with other health problems, like heart issues, weak bones, or kidney problems. Eating the right foods can help you manage these other conditions and keep your body healthy.

4. Managing Energy and Weight: One of the main symptoms of lupus is feeling really tired, but eating a balanced diet can help give you more energy. Eating foods that keep your blood sugar steady can also help prevent weight gain, which can make you feel even more tired.

Foods to Include and Avoid

What you eat can either help or hurt your lupus symptoms. While everyone's body is different, there are some general rules that can help you make better food choices.

Foods to Include:

1. Fruits and Vegetables: These are packed with vitamins, minerals, and fiber that help fight inflammation. Brightly colored fruits and veggies are especially helpful, so eat lots of spinach, carrots, berries, and apples. Dark leafy greens like spinach and kale are also really good for your immune system.

2. Omega-3 Fatty Acids: Omega-3s, found in fish like salmon, can help reduce inflammation. If you don't eat fish, you can get omega-3s from things like chia seeds, walnuts, and flaxseeds.

3. Whole Grains: Whole grains, like brown rice and oatmeal, are healthy foods that help give you energy and keep your blood sugar levels steady.

4. Lean Proteins: Foods like chicken, turkey, tofu, and beans help build and repair muscles, give you energy, and support your immune system.

5. Healthy Fats: Healthy fats like those in olive oil, avocado, and nuts help reduce inflammation and keep you energized.

6. Calcium and Vitamin D: If you're taking certain medications for lupus, they can weaken your bones. Foods

like milk, yogurt, and leafy greens can help keep your bones strong, and getting vitamin D from foods or sunlight is important too.

Foods to Avoid:

1. Processed Foods: Fast food, sugary snacks, and packaged foods are high in unhealthy fats and sugars. These foods can make inflammation worse and add extra calories, which can make you feel more tired.

2. Saturated Fats and Trans Fats: Foods like fatty meats, butter, and fried foods are full of unhealthy fats that can increase inflammation and hurt your

heart. Try to avoid these foods whenever you can.

3. Salt: Too much salt can cause your body to hold onto extra water, raise your blood pressure, and put stress on your kidneys. It's a good idea to cut back on salt and use herbs or lemon to flavor your food instead.

4. Nightshade Vegetables: Some people with lupus find that certain vegetables like tomatoes, potatoes, and peppers can make their symptoms worse. If this happens to you, try cutting them out for a while and see if it helps.

5. Alcohol: Alcohol can interfere with some lupus medications and can also cause inflammation in your body. It's best to limit alcohol or avoid it altogether.

Supplements and Nutritional Support

While eating the right foods is important, some people with lupus may also need extra help from supplements. Supplements can give you the nutrients you need if you're not getting enough from food.

1. Omega-3 Supplements: If you don't eat enough fish, you can take omega-3

supplements to help reduce inflammation.

2. Vitamin D: People with lupus often don't get enough vitamin D, which is important for bone health. A vitamin D supplement might help.

3. Calcium: If you're taking medications like steroids, your bones may become weaker. Calcium supplements can help keep your bones strong.

4. Probiotics: Probiotics are good bacteria that help with digestion and overall immune health. You can get them from yogurt or as supplements.

5. Antioxidants: Antioxidants, like vitamin C and vitamin E, can protect your body from damage and help reduce inflammation.

Conclusion

Eating the right foods is one of the best ways to manage lupus. A diet full of fruits, vegetables, lean proteins, healthy fats, and calcium-rich foods can help reduce inflammation, support your immune system, and keep you feeling energized. Avoiding processed foods, unhealthy fats, salt, and alcohol can help prevent flare-ups. Some supplements, like omega-3s, vitamin D, and calcium, can also give you extra support. Always talk to your doctor before making big changes to your diet or adding new supplements, but remember that fueling your body with the right foods can help you feel your best and manage lupus better.

CHAPTER 8: EXERCISE AND PHYSICAL ACTIVITY WITH LUPUS

Lupus is a condition where the body's immune system attacks its own healthy cells, causing symptoms like tiredness, joint pain, and swelling. Even though managing lupus can be tough, staying active through exercise is an important part of staying healthy. Exercise can help reduce pain, improve mood, and manage symptoms. In this chapter, we'll look at the benefits of exercise, how to choose the right routine, and how to stay safe when exercising during a flare-up.

Benefits of Staying Active

Exercise can help people with lupus feel better in many ways:

1. Reduces Pain and Stiffness: Exercise can make your muscles and joints more flexible, which helps reduce stiffness and improve movement. It can also ease the pain that comes with lupus in the joints.

2. Improves Mood: Dealing with lupus can sometimes make people feel sad or stressed. Exercise releases chemicals in

the brain called endorphins that make you feel happy and reduce feelings of sadness and worry.

3. Keeps Your Heart Healthy: People with lupus have a higher chance of developing heart problems, so exercise helps make your heart stronger and improves blood circulation.

4. Boosts Energy: Even though lupus can make you feel tired, exercise actually helps increase your energy levels, making you feel less tired throughout the day.

5. Helps Maintain a Healthy Weight: Staying active helps keep your weight

healthy. This is important because being a healthy weight reduces strain on your joints and lowers the risk of getting other health problems, like diabetes.

6. Improves Sleep: Exercise helps you sleep better at night. When you get better sleep, you feel more rested and have more energy during the day.

Choosing the Right Exercise Routine

It's important to choose an exercise routine that works for you and feels good. Here are some tips:

1. Start Slow: If you're new to exercise, start with simple activities and slowly work your way up as you get stronger.

2. Pick Low-Impact Exercises: Since lupus can cause joint pain, low-impact exercises are best because they are easier on your joints. Some good examples include:

Walking

Swimming

Cycling

Yoga

Pilates

Using an elliptical machine

3. Try Strength Training: Strength training helps build muscle and prevent bone loss, which can happen from lupus medications. You can use light weights or resistance bands to strengthen your muscles without putting too much stress on your joints.

4. Stretch and Improve Flexibility: Stretching exercises help keep your muscles flexible, reduce stiffness, and prevent injury. Yoga and Pilates are good options because they mix stretching and strength-building.

5. Set Realistic Goals: When starting, set small, achievable goals. Don't push yourself too hard—listen to your body. You can increase the time and difficulty of your workouts as you feel stronger.

6. Talk to Your Doctor: Before starting any new exercise routine, ask your doctor for advice. They can help you choose exercises that are safe and right for your symptoms.

How to Exercise Safely During a Flare-Up

A flare-up happens when lupus symptoms, like joint pain and swelling, get worse. Even when you're having a flare-up, you can still exercise safely. Here's how:

1. Listen to Your Body: The most important rule is to pay attention to how your body feels. If you feel pain, stop. It's important to know the difference between normal muscle tiredness and pain caused by lupus. If you feel pain, take a break and talk to your doctor if needed.

2. Do Gentle Exercises: During a flare-up, stick to easy exercises like walking, stretching, or yoga. Avoid intense workouts that could stress your joints.

3. Exercise in Shorter Sessions: Instead of doing a long workout, break it into shorter sessions. You could take a 10-minute walk in the morning, afternoon, and evening. This way, you still stay active without overdoing it.

4. Warm Up and Cool Down: It's important to warm up before you exercise and cool down afterward. Spend a few minutes stretching gently to prepare your muscles and to relax them after your workout.

5. Drink Water: Dehydration can make lupus symptoms worse, so be sure to drink plenty of water before, during, and after exercising.

6. Rest When Needed: If you're feeling really tired or your symptoms are getting worse, it's okay to take a rest. Pushing yourself too hard can make things worse.

7. Adjust Activities if Needed: If an exercise hurts during a flare-up, you can modify it. For example, you might change a yoga pose to make it more comfortable. Don't be afraid to adapt exercises to fit what your body needs.

Conclusion

Exercise is an important way to manage lupus and stay healthy. It can reduce pain, improve mood, boost energy, and keep your heart and bones strong. When choosing an exercise routine, focus on low-impact activities and strength training. During a flare-up, listen to your body and choose gentle exercises to avoid injury. Always talk to your doctor before starting a new routine, and remember to be consistent and patient with yourself. By exercising safely and finding a routine that works for you, you can live well with lupus.

CHAPTER 9: EMOTIONAL HEALTH AND COPING WITH LUPUS

Lupus is a disease that affects not only the body but also your mind and emotions. The pain, tiredness, and swelling caused by lupus are often the main focus, but the mental and emotional challenges are just as important. Many people with lupus experience anxiety, sadness, and frustration because the disease can be unpredictable and hard to manage. In this chapter, we'll talk about how lupus can affect your feelings, ways to cope with anxiety and depression, and how to build a support system of people who can help you.

The Mental and Emotional Impact of Lupus

Lupus can affect more than just your body. It can also make you feel stressed or sad. Here are some ways lupus can impact your emotions:

1. The Stress of Uncertainty: Lupus can be unpredictable. Sometimes your symptoms get better, and sometimes they get worse without warning. This can make you feel anxious because you never know when your symptoms will

come back. It can also make you feel helpless or frustrated.

2. Tiredness and "Brain Fog": Many people with lupus feel extremely tired all the time, even after sleeping. This tiredness can make it hard to focus or think clearly. It can also make daily tasks harder, which might make you feel sad or left out of activities.

3. Feeling Alone: Sometimes, people with lupus can feel isolated because they can't do all the things they used to enjoy, like hanging out with friends. This can lead to loneliness and make you feel like you don't belong.

4. Body Changes: Lupus can cause skin rashes, hair loss, and other visible changes. This can affect how you feel about your appearance and might make you feel self-conscious or depressed.

5. Fear of the Future: Because lupus can be unpredictable, you might worry about what will happen in the future. You may wonder if your symptoms will get worse or how lupus will affect your life later on.

Coping with Anxiety and Depression

It's normal to feel anxious or sad when you have lupus, but there are ways to cope with these feelings. Here are some helpful strategies:

1. Acknowledge Your Feelings: It's important to recognize and accept that it's okay to feel anxious or sad. Your emotions are valid, and taking care of your mental health is just as important as taking care of your body.

2. Practice Relaxation: Techniques like deep breathing, meditation, or muscle relaxation can help reduce stress. Taking just a few minutes each day to focus on your breathing or relax your muscles can help you feel calmer.

3. Exercise: Moving your body, like walking, swimming, or doing yoga, can

improve both your body and mind. Exercise releases "feel-good" chemicals in the brain that can boost your mood and help reduce stress.

4. Set Realistic Goals: With lupus, it's important to adjust your expectations. You may need to take more breaks or ask for help. By setting small goals, you can feel proud of your achievements, even if they are small.

5. Talk to a Therapist: Talking to a counselor can help you work through your feelings. A therapist can help you understand your emotions and teach you ways to deal with them.

6. Medication: Sometimes, medication is needed to help with feelings of anxiety or depression. If your emotions are interfering with your daily life, talk to your doctor about the possibility of using medication.

7. Journaling: Writing down your thoughts and feelings can help you understand and process them. It's a way to express yourself without worrying about what others think.

Building a Support System

Having people around you who understand what you're going through is very important for your emotional well-being. Here are some ways to build your support system:

1. Talk to Family and Friends: Share how you feel with people close to you. Let them know what you're going through and how they can support you. It's important to have people who listen and care about your well-being.

2. Join a Support Group: Talking to other people with lupus can help you feel less alone. A support group is a place where you can share your experiences and learn from others. Whether it's in person or online, support groups can make you feel understood.

3. Communicate with Your Doctors: Be open with your healthcare team about how you're feeling emotionally. They can offer support, suggest resources, or adjust your treatment plan to address both your physical and emotional health.

4. Stay Engaged: Even if lupus limits some activities, it's important to stay involved in things that make you happy. Hobbies, volunteering, or spending time with people can help you feel connected and give you a sense of purpose.

5. Get Professional Help: If your emotions become too overwhelming, seeking professional help can provide

relief. A therapist can guide you through your feelings and teach you ways to feel better.

Conclusion

Living with lupus can be difficult, and it's important to take care of your mental health just as much as your physical health. By recognizing your emotions, finding ways to cope with anxiety and sadness, and building a strong support system, you can improve your emotional well-being. Remember, it's okay to feel what you're feeling, and there are many people and resources to help you along the way.

CHAPTER 10: THE ROLE OF YOUR HEALTHCARE TEAM

Lupus is a serious illness that can affect many parts of your body, making it tricky to manage. One of the most important things you can do is to work closely with a team of doctors who understand lupus and can help you feel better. This chapter will explain why it's important to have a good relationship with your doctors, how to create a plan for managing your lupus, and when it might be helpful to get a second opinion.

Why Working with Your Doctors is Important

When you have lupus, you'll likely have a team of doctors who help you with different parts of the disease. Since lupus can affect many organs in your body, you might need different types of doctors, such as a rheumatologist (who focuses on autoimmune diseases), a heart doctor, or a skin doctor. It's important to work closely with all these doctors to get the best care.

Here's why it's so important to work with your doctors:

1. Complete Care: Since lupus affects many parts of your body, you need

different doctors to help manage all of these problems. For example, a rheumatologist can help with the immune system, while a heart doctor can help with any heart issues.

2. Personalized Treatment: Everyone with lupus experiences it differently. By talking with your doctors, you can make a treatment plan that works just for you. Your doctors will listen to your symptoms and goals and create a plan that helps you the most.

3. Better Decisions: The more you communicate with your doctors, the better the treatment can be. Asking questions and being open about how

you feel helps your doctors give you the best advice and treatment.

4. Catching Problems Early: Sometimes lupus can cause problems in your organs that you don't feel right away. By working with your doctors, they can do tests to check for issues before they get serious.

5. Ongoing Care: Lupus can flare up at any time, so it's important to keep track of how you feel and adjust your treatment plan if needed. Your doctors will help you stay on top of your condition.

How to Build a Good Care Plan

Creating a care plan for lupus is something you do with your doctors. It should not only include medicine but also consider your lifestyle, how you're feeling emotionally, and what you want in your life. Here's how you can create a good care plan:

1. Set Goals: The first step in making a care plan is to decide what you want to achieve, like reducing flare-ups, feeling more energetic, or managing pain. Your doctors can help you set these goals and make a plan to reach them.

2. Regular Check-ups: Since lupus can affect many organs, it's important to have regular tests to check for any new problems. Your care plan should include when you need these tests so you can catch any issues early.

3. Managing Medications: Medicines are a big part of lupus treatment, but it can take time to find the right ones. Your care plan should tell you exactly when and how to take each medicine and what to do if the medicine isn't working or if it has side effects.

4. Healthy Lifestyle: Eating healthy food and exercising can help with lupus symptoms. Although there is no special diet for lupus, eating well and staying

active can make you feel better. Your doctors may refer you to a nutritionist or physical therapist to help create a plan that works for you.

5. Mental Health: Lupus can also affect your emotions. Feeling sad, anxious, or stressed is common for people with lupus. It's important to include emotional health in your care plan. Your doctors might suggest seeing a counselor or joining a support group.

6. Emergency Plan: Sometimes, lupus can cause sudden serious problems that need immediate attention, like a high fever or severe pain. Your care plan should include what to do if something like this happens, so you're prepared.

When to Get a Second Opinion

Sometimes, you might feel unsure about your diagnosis or treatment, and that's okay. If you feel like your current treatment isn't working, or if you just want to know more about your options, getting a second opinion might help. Here are some times when getting another doctor's opinion can be helpful:

1. Not Sure About Your Diagnosis: If you're not sure whether you have lupus or if you think your doctor might be wrong, getting a second opinion can help. Sometimes, lupus symptoms are similar to other illnesses, so it's important to be sure.

2. Treatment Isn't Working: If the medicine or treatment your doctor gave you isn't helping, or if it's causing too many side effects, it might be time to get a second opinion. Another doctor might suggest different treatments that work better for you.

3. Conflicting Advice: If different doctors are giving you different advice, it can be confusing. A second opinion can help you make sense of the choices and decide what's best for you.

4. Complex Cases: Lupus can sometimes cause very serious problems. If your lupus is affecting

many parts of your body, it might help to see a specialist or a doctor who knows a lot about lupus.

5. Feeling Uncomfortable: You should feel comfortable with your doctor. If you don't feel like your doctor is listening to you, or if you don't trust their advice, getting a second opinion might help you feel more confident in your treatment.

Conclusion

Your healthcare team is a big part of living well with lupus. By working together with your doctors, making a good care plan, and knowing when to ask for another opinion, you can take control of your lupus and live a better life. Remember that your doctors are there to help, and it's okay to ask questions and ask for help whenever you need it.

CHAPTER 11: PREGNANCY AND LUPUS

Pregnancy is a special time, but it can be more complicated if you have lupus. Lupus is a disease where your immune system mistakenly attacks your own body, and it can affect many different organs. This chapter will explain how to manage lupus during pregnancy, the risks that mothers with lupus might face, and things to think about after giving birth.

Managing Lupus During Pregnancy

If you're pregnant and have lupus, you'll need extra care to keep yourself and your baby healthy. Many women with lupus can have a successful pregnancy, but it's important to manage the disease well to reduce the risk of complications. Here are some important tips:

1. Work with Your Doctors: It's really important to have both an obstetrician (a doctor for pregnancy) and a rheumatologist (a doctor for lupus) working together to take care of you. Your doctors will help manage your lupus and make sure your baby is healthy.

2. Watch for Flare-Ups: Lupus can get worse during pregnancy, and flare-ups are possible. If you feel like your lupus is getting worse, contact your doctors right away. They can change your treatment to help keep things under control.

3. Medication: Some medications that help treat lupus are safe during pregnancy, like corticosteroids and hydroxychloroquine. But other medicines, like methotrexate, should be avoided. Your doctors will help you find the right medications to take while you're pregnant.

4. Regular Checkups: During pregnancy, you'll need lots of checkups

to make sure both you and your baby are doing well. This might include blood tests, ultrasounds, and other monitoring to watch for complications.

5. Healthy Lifestyle: Eating a balanced diet, getting plenty of rest, staying hydrated, and managing stress are all really important during pregnancy. Light exercise, as advised by your doctors, can also help keep you healthy.

Risks and Precautions for Expecting Mothers

Pregnancy can be more risky for women with lupus. It's important to be aware of these risks so you can take steps to stay healthy:

1. Flare-Ups: Women with lupus may have flare-ups during pregnancy, especially in the first two trimesters. These flare-ups can affect your organs and might even cause preterm birth. Keeping lupus under control is important to avoid complications.

2. Preterm Birth and Low Birth Weight: Women with lupus are more likely to give birth early or have a baby who is smaller than usual. Preterm babies may have trouble breathing or feeding, so it's important to closely monitor your pregnancy.

3. Preeclampsia: This is a serious condition where you have high blood pressure and can damage your organs. Women with lupus are more likely to get preeclampsia, so regular blood pressure checks are really important.

4. Miscarriage: There's a slightly higher risk of miscarriage for women with lupus, especially if the disease is active. But with proper care, many women with lupus have successful pregnancies.

5. Blood Clots: Lupus can increase the risk of blood clots, which can be dangerous. Your doctor may suggest blood thinners to help prevent clots during pregnancy.

6. Antiphospholipid Syndrome (APS): Some women with lupus also have APS, which makes blood clots more likely. If you have APS, your doctor may prescribe medicines to reduce the risk of clots.

Postpartum Considerations for Lupus Patients

The time after childbirth, called the postpartum period, can also be challenging for women with lupus. Here are some things to consider:

1. Flare-Ups After Birth: After giving birth, many women with lupus

experience flare-ups. This can happen because of the stress of childbirth, hormonal changes, or lack of sleep. Let your doctors know if you feel worse after giving birth.

2. Breastfeeding: If you want to breastfeed, make sure your doctor knows what medications you're taking. Some lupus medicines are safe for breastfeeding, like hydroxychloroquine and corticosteroids, but always check with your doctor before taking any medication.

3. Postpartum Depression: Many women feel sad or overwhelmed after having a baby, and women with lupus may be at higher risk for postpartum

depression. If you feel depressed, talk to your doctor for support and help.

4. Fatigue: It's normal to feel tired after having a baby, and if you have lupus, you might feel even more tired. Rest, accepting help from others, and being patient with yourself will help you recover.

5. Contraception: After giving birth, talk to your doctor about birth control if you're not planning to have another baby right away. Some birth control options might not be safe for women with lupus, so make sure you choose one that works for you.

Conclusion

Pregnancy with lupus needs extra care, but many women with lupus can have healthy pregnancies. By working closely with your doctors, managing flare-ups, and staying on top of your health, you can give yourself and your baby the best chance for a safe pregnancy and postpartum period. Always talk to your doctors to make sure you're making the right decisions for your health and your baby's health.

CHAPTER 12: LUPUS AND WORK

Lupus is a disease where the body's immune system attacks its own cells, which can make everyday activities, including work, harder. It can cause things like fatigue, joint pain, headaches, and skin rashes. Even though lupus can make working difficult, many people with lupus still work by finding ways to manage their symptoms. In this chapter, we'll talk about how to balance work with lupus, how to talk to your boss about your condition, and what legal protections you have at work.

Navigating Work with Lupus

Balancing work and lupus can be tricky because everyone experiences the disease differently. Some people might have mild symptoms, while others might struggle more. Here are some tips for managing work with lupus:

1. Listen to Your Body: It's important to pay attention to how your body feels. If you're tired, in pain, or having other symptoms, don't push yourself too hard. Knowing when to take a break is key to avoiding making your symptoms worse.

2. Set Realistic Expectations: With lupus, it's okay to adjust your workload. You may need to change your hours or ask for help with tasks if you're feeling tired or unwell. Be realistic about what you can handle to prevent burning out.

3. Time Management: Managing your time is very important. Break down big tasks into smaller steps so you don't get overwhelmed. Using planners or apps can help you stay organized and reduce stress.

4. Take Breaks: It's important to take regular breaks at work. This can help you avoid feeling too tired or having a flare-up. If you sit for long periods, try

to stand up or walk around for a few minutes every hour.

5. Stay Hydrated and Eat Healthily: Drinking enough water and eating healthy foods can help keep your energy up and prevent lupus symptoms from getting worse.

6. Practice Stress Management: Stress can make lupus worse, so it's important to find ways to relax. Try things like deep breathing, meditation, or taking a walk to help reduce stress at work.

Communicating with Your Employer

Talking to your boss about your lupus is important, but it can also feel difficult. Here are some ways to communicate with your employer:

1. Be Honest but Keep Some Privacy: You don't have to share everything about your lupus, but it's helpful to let your boss know you have a health condition that can make you tired or affect your work sometimes. It's up to you how much you want to share.

2. Ask for Reasonable Accommodations: If lupus is making it hard for you to do your job, you can

ask for changes at work, like flexible hours or the ability to work from home. These changes are called accommodations and can help you stay productive without making your symptoms worse.

3. Be Ready for Questions: Your boss might ask you how lupus affects your work. You don't have to share personal details, but explaining how it can impact your day and suggesting ways to help can make things easier. For example, you might ask for more breaks or a different schedule if needed.

4. Keep Your Employer Updated: If you have a flare-up or need time off, let

your employer know as soon as possible. Keeping them informed helps you get the support you need and shows you are working to manage your health.

5. Have a Plan for Time Off: Sometimes, you might need time off for doctor visits or to rest during a flare-up. It's good to have a plan in place for how to take sick leave or get help with your tasks when you need time off.

Legal Rights and Protections for Lupus Patients

As a person with lupus, there are laws that protect you at work. Here are some important protections you should know about:

1. Americans with Disabilities Act (ADA): The ADA is a law that helps people with disabilities, including lupus, by making sure they are treated fairly at work. It requires employers to provide reasonable accommodations, like allowing flexible hours or working from home, if needed.

2. Family and Medical Leave Act (FMLA): If your lupus symptoms get worse and you need to take time off, the FMLA allows you to take up to 12 weeks of unpaid leave each year. Your job is protected, meaning you can't be fired for taking this time off to take care of your health.

3. Disability Benefits: If you're unable to work for a while due to lupus, you may be able to get financial support through short-term or long-term disability insurance. Check with your employer to find out if this is an option.

4. State Laws: In addition to federal laws, your state might have extra protections for people with disabilities,

so it's a good idea to learn about your state's specific laws to understand your rights.

Conclusion

Balancing lupus with work is challenging, but it's possible with the right strategies and support. By listening to your body, communicating with your employer, and knowing your legal rights, you can find ways to manage both your job and your health. With time and careful planning, you can continue to work while taking care of yourself.

CHAPTER 13: LOOKING AHEAD

Living with lupus can be tough, but with the right care, it's possible to manage the disease and lead a full, happy life. In this chapter, we will talk about how to set goals for your health, prevent problems, and keep a positive attitude to help you live your best life.

Setting Goals for Your Health Journey

Setting goals is an important part of managing lupus. Having clear goals can help you stay motivated and focused on getting better. Here are some ways to set goals that will work for you:

1. Create Personal Health Goals: Think about what you want to achieve with your health. This could be feeling less tired, controlling pain in your joints, or eating healthier. Make sure your goals are specific and measurable, like "I will reduce my joint pain by 30% in the next three months by exercising and taking my medicine."

2. Set Short-Term and Long-Term Goals: Short-term goals help you stay on track and give you quick wins. For example, a short-term goal might be to visit your doctor regularly. A long-term goal could be staying healthy for many

years or achieving a certain fitness level.

3. Track Your Progress: Keep track of your progress. You can use a journal or an app to monitor how you feel, what medicines you take, how you eat, and how much exercise you do. This helps you see your improvements and make changes if needed.

4. Celebrate Small Wins: Every little success is important. Whether it's sticking to your treatment plan, feeling better, or just getting through a tough day, take time to recognize what you've accomplished.

5. Work with Your Healthcare Team: Your doctor and other healthcare providers are there to help you. Work with them to set goals that match your health needs.

Preventing Complications and Managing Risks

Lupus can cause problems in your body, but you can prevent many issues by being careful. Here are some tips to help you stay healthy:

1. Follow Your Treatment Plan: Take your medicines as your doctor says and go to your appointments. Medicines like steroids and other treatments help control lupus and prevent flare-ups.

2. Take Care of Your Organs: Lupus can affect your kidneys, heart, and other organs. Make sure your doctor checks how your organs are doing by doing regular tests like blood pressure or kidney function checks.

3. Avoid Infections: Since lupus and its treatments can weaken your immune system, infections are a risk. Wash your hands often, avoid sick people, and talk to your doctor about vaccines to keep you safe.

4. Stay Healthy: A healthy lifestyle can help you avoid problems and manage lupus better. This includes:

Eating a balanced diet: Eat lots of fruits, vegetables, whole grains, and lean proteins, and avoid processed foods.

Exercise: Regular exercise helps your joints, reduces tiredness, and lifts your mood. Activities like walking, swimming, or yoga are great options.

Sleep: Getting enough rest helps your body heal. Aim for 7-9 hours of sleep each night.

5. Know Your Body: Pay attention to any changes in how you feel. If you notice something unusual or a flare-up of symptoms, talk to your doctor right away to prevent problems.

Embracing a Positive Outlook and Living Your Best Life

Lupus may bring challenges, but keeping a positive mindset can help you handle the difficulties. A good attitude doesn't mean ignoring the tough parts, but it can help you feel more in control and ready to live a full life. Here are some tips to stay positive:

1. Focus on What You Can Control: You can't control lupus, but you can control how you take care of your health. Stay active, eat well, and follow your treatment plan. Doing these things helps you feel strong and in charge.

2. Build a Support System: It's important to have people who support you. This can be family, friends, or people who understand lupus. They can help you with tasks, listen to you, or just be there when you need them.

3. Take Time for Yourself: Do things that make you happy and help you relax. Whether it's reading a book, listening to music, or spending time outdoors, taking care of your mind is just as important as taking care of your body.

4. Celebrate Life: Even with lupus, you can still enjoy life. Spend time with the people you care about, do activities you love, and celebrate the good moments.

5. Stay Resilient: Living with lupus takes strength. There will be hard days, but remember that every day is a new chance to move forward. Resilience helps you keep going even when things are tough.

Conclusion

Managing lupus isn't just about controlling symptoms—it's about setting goals, preventing problems, and keeping a positive outlook on life. By making healthy choices, working with your healthcare team, and focusing on the good things, you can live a happy, full life despite the challenges of lupus. You are not alone, and with the right attitude and support, you can keep moving forward and thriving.

Thank You!

As we reach the end of this journey together, I want to take a moment to express my deepest gratitude to you, the reader. Writing this book, Lupus Uncovered: Essential Insights and Practical Guidance for Patients, has been a labor of love, and knowing that you are here, reading these words, is truly humbling. Whether you're living with lupus yourself, supporting a loved one, or simply seeking information, your interest in this topic shows your commitment to better understanding the disease and its impact on lives.

A Personal Note

Before we conclude, I want to share a personal note of appreciation. Lupus, as many of you know, is a chronic disease that often requires constant care, attention, and, at times, a heavy emotional toll. As someone who has spent years researching and reflecting on lupus through the lens of both a patient and a caregiver, I have seen firsthand how life can be profoundly altered by the disease. In my own experience, I have encountered countless moments of doubt and difficulty. But I've also witnessed the remarkable strength and resilience of individuals who, despite the challenges, continue to push forward.

Through this book, I hope to have provided you with not only the medical knowledge and practical advice necessary to live well with lupus but also the encouragement and emotional support you may need to stay motivated and positive. Whether you're just beginning your journey or have been managing lupus for years, remember that you are not alone. The community of lupus patients, caregivers, and healthcare professionals is vast, and together we can learn, share, and grow.

The Power of Knowledge

When you're diagnosed with lupus, it often feels as if the world has suddenly shifted beneath your feet. There are many unknowns, and it's easy to feel overwhelmed by the complexity of the disease. Throughout this book, I've aimed to break down the complexities of lupus into manageable, digestible pieces. From understanding the medical aspects of lupus, such as how it affects the immune system, to learning practical tips on managing symptoms and building a supportive care team, my goal has always been to empower you with knowledge.

Education is one of the most important tools you have when managing any chronic illness, and lupus is no exception. The more you know about your condition, the more confident and proactive you can be in your healthcare. Lupus may be unpredictable, but with a deeper understanding, you can better anticipate the ups and downs and take control of the aspects you can influence.

Acknowledging the Challenges

That being said, lupus is not an easy condition to live with. It's important to acknowledge the emotional and physical toll that comes with the disease. From flare-ups and fatigue to the mental strain of navigating the healthcare system, the journey can feel daunting at times. But one of the most important lessons I've learned, and that I hope you take away from this book, is that even in the face of adversity, there are ways to manage, adapt, and thrive.

As we discussed in earlier chapters, setting achievable goals, adopting a healthy lifestyle, and building a supportive network of people are critical steps in living well with lupus. These strategies, while not always easy to implement, can make all the difference in maintaining a sense of control, empowerment, and hope. And remember, setbacks are a part of life—if you have a difficult day, or even a challenging week or month, don't be too hard on yourself. It's important to show yourself the same kindness and patience that you would offer to a loved one.

The Importance of Community and Support

One of the most powerful things about living with a chronic illness is the sense of community that exists among those who share similar experiences. You are not isolated in your journey. Whether it's a support group, online forums, or the encouragement you receive from family and friends, these connections are invaluable. The people around you—whether they are fellow lupus patients, caregivers, or healthcare providers—form a network that can help you navigate the ups and downs of this disease.

I want to take a moment to thank all of the lupus warriors out there, each one of you who shares your story, your struggles, and your triumphs. Your courage in facing lupus head-on inspires me every day, and I'm sure it inspires others as well. If there's one thing I've learned, it's that the more we share, the more we help each other. Your experiences, whether in person or through digital platforms, help create a broader understanding of what it truly means to live with lupus.

Looking Forward

As we wrap up this book, I want to leave you with one final thought: while lupus is a challenging disease, it is also a journey that can be filled with resilience, hope, and strength. The path may not always be easy, but it is possible to live a fulfilling life despite the obstacles. The goal is not perfection, but progress. Small steps forward, each day, add up to a significant difference in the quality of life you can achieve.

Whether you're facing lupus yourself or caring for someone who is, remember that the power of knowledge, the strength of community, and the importance of self-care are always there to help you along the way. Thank you for taking the time to read this book. I hope the information, stories, and advice shared here help guide you on your journey to living well with lupus.

And most importantly, thank you for being part of this shared community of lupus warriors. You are not alone, and together, we can continue to uncover the best ways to thrive with lupus.

With gratitude and hope,

Pete Gregory

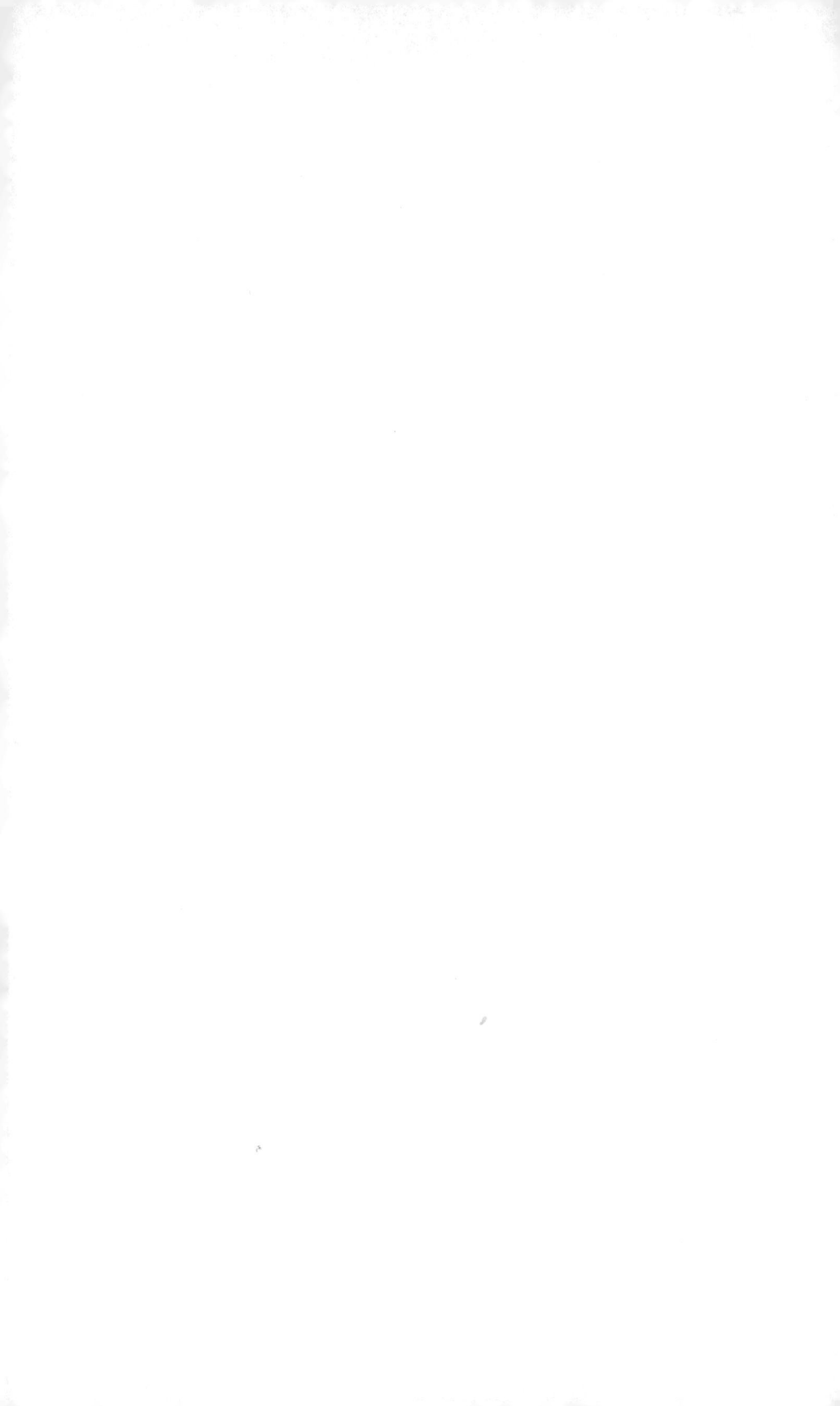

Made in the USA
Columbia, SC
05 July 2025